All About
Pressure Ulcers and Positioning

By Laura Flynn R.N., B.N., M.B.A., In consultation with her nurse educator associates and physicians who assisted in contributing and editing.

Thanks also to the following organizations: Canadian Association for Wound Care (CAWC), National Pressure Ulcer Advisory Board (NPUAP), Wound Ostomy Continence Nurses (WOCN) association, The Agency for Health Care Policy (AHCPR) and the Royal Ontario Nurses Association of Ontario (RNAO) for their reference of Long Term Care (LTC) positioning guidelines.

ISBN No: 978 1 896616 84 1 © 2014 Mediscript Communications Inc.

Pressure Ulcers. Prevention of Pressure Ulcers. Positioning and Pressure Ulcers. Self Study Guide for Positioning and Pressure Ulcers.

The publisher, Mediscript Communications Inc., acknowledges the financial support of the Government of Canada through the Canadian Book Fund for our publishing activities.

www.mediscript.net

Printed in Canada

Book and Front Cover design by:
Brian Adamson, www.AdamsonGraphics.net

PUP1002010

CONTENTS

Medical Chart Bloopers

- On the 2nd day the knee was better and on the 3rd day it disappeared completely.

- Skin: Somewhat pale but present.

- The patient is tearful and crying constantly. She also appears to be depressed.

- Occasional, constant, infrequent headaches.

- Patient has chest pain if she lies on her left side for over a year.

Source: www.nursefriendly.com

Chapter 1
INTRODUCTION

This book provides basic, non controversial, and trusted information that can help a wide spectrum of readers.

The primary objective of the information is to help the reader provide effective quality care to a loved one or someone in his or her care.

Conversely a person at risk for developing a pressure ulcer or already suffering from a pressure ulcer can be better informed and comply and assist more effectively in treatment and prevention by reading this book.

All the information is reliable and was written by a group of eminent nurse educators who ensured the information complies with best practice guidelines and satisfies the various accreditation and regulatory bodies. In fact, there is so much unreliable information on the internet, these "All About" publications are HON (Health On the Net) certified.

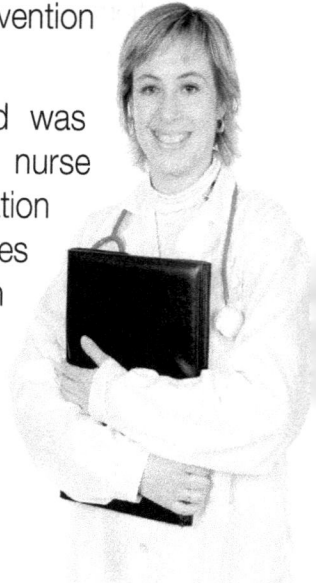

Consequently this book can be an invaluable aid to:

- A caregiver caring for a relative or someone in the family.
- A health worker seeking a reference aid.
- A patient or person at risk for pressure ulcers or currently suffering from one.
- A person involved in health care wishing to expand his or her knowledge of pressure ulcers.

SOMETHING TO THINK ABOUT...

That man is blest who does his best

and leaves the rest; do not worry.

Charles F. Deems

AN IMPORTANT MESSAGE FROM THE PUBLISHER

Each person's treatment, advice, medical aids, physical therapy and other approaches to health care are unique and highly dependant upon the diagnosis and overall assessment by the medical team.

We emphasize therefore that the information within this book is not a substitute for the advice and treatment from a health care professional.

This book provides generic information concerning the disease process and common sense well established care practices for preventing, treating and positioning pressure ulcer sufferers or at risk people.

With all this in mind, the publishers and authors disclaim any responsibility for any adverse effects resulting directly or indirectly from the suggestions contained within this book or from any misunderstanding of the content on the part of the reader.

WHAT DO YOU KNOW

It helps to figure out how much you know before starting. In this way you will have an idea as to the gaps in your knowledge prior to reading the content. Please circle to indicate the best answer. Remember, at this stage, you are not expected to know all the answers:

1. Tissue damage can occur when someone being cared for slides down in a chair. The injury occurs because of:

a) Friction

b) Shear

c) Advanced age

d) Posture

2. To prevent pressure ulcers for people who use a wheelchair, you should:

a) Assist with a position change every 15 minutes

b) Assist with a position change every 2 hours

c) Provide a donut-shaped cushion for the wheelchair

d) Avoid any special cushion as they are not effective in relieving or reducing pressure

3. The side-lying position is called:

a) Supine

b) Lateral

c) Prone

d) Sim's

4. What is a contracture?

a) Abnormal shortening of a muscle

b) The small bone at the end of the spinal column

c) The force that occurs when one object is rubbed against another

d) An area where the bone sticks out from the flat surface of the body

5. What is the estimated annual cost of pressure ulcer care in the U.S. each year?

a) 1.5 million dollars

b) Over 50 billion dollars

c) Between 5 and 8.5 billion dollars

d) There are no estimates for the overall cost

6. Which score on the Braden Scale indicates the highest risk of pressure ulcer development?

a) 7

b) 10

c) 13

d) 16

7. Which position is not recommended for clients with breathing or spinal problems?

a) Fowler's

b) Prone

c) Lateral

d) Supine

ANSWERS

1. b) "Shear" is the name for this type of physical damage that can contribute to a pressure ulcer forming.

2. a) A frequent change of position – ideally, every 15 minutes – can help prevent pressure ulcers from forming.

3. b) Lateral is the correct term for the side-lying position. The others will be explained in Chapter 5.

4. a) A contracture, or abnormal shortening of a muscle, can be caused by inactivity, eg. prolonged bed rest.

5. c) The annual cost is between 5 and 8.5 billion dollars and growing.

6. a) The lower the score the higher the risk, so the correct answer is 7.

7. b) The prone position – lying flat on one's front – is not recommended for these people.

PRESSURE ULCERS
AND POSITIONING

Have you ever cared for someone with a pressure ulcer? Pressure ulcers can seriously affect a person's health. They can cause physical pain and emotional stress for sufferers and their families. They lead to longer stays in the hospital or nursing home. They can interfere with recovery. Anyone who must stay in a bed or a chair for prolonged periods of time is at risk for developing pressure ulcers. Other factors also increase the risk for pressure ulcers.

Luckily, most pressure ulcers can be prevented. As a caregiver you have a vital role in preventing pressure ulcers. This book provides you with information about pressure ulcers and how to prevent them.

WORDS YOU SHOULD KNOW

Bed cradle

A device that helps keep the bed linens from touching the client's feet

Body alignment

Alignment refers to positioning. Good body alignment means making sure that limbs and joints are properly positioned and supported.

Bony prominence

An area where the bone sticks out from the flat surface of the body. Examples are the tailbone, heel, ankles, shoulders, hips and elbows. These areas are especially prone to pressure ulcers.

Coccyx

Small bone at the end of the spinal column

Contracture

Abnormal shortening of a muscle. The muscle becomes resistant to stretching, making movement of the muscle difficult. A contracture can lead to a permanent disability.

Footboard

A footboard is a board placed at the foot of the bed so that the client's feet can be positioned against it. It is important that the feet are placed flat against the footboard. A footboard helps to prevent footdrop.

Footdrop

The toes drop and point downwards due to muscle weakness. Footdrop can lead to a permanent disability.

Friction

The force that occurs when one object is rubbed against another object

Mortality

The death rate

Prevalence

The number of cases of a condition within a certain population at a given point in time

Sacrum

A large triangular bone at the back part of the pelvis

Shear

A parallel force that may cause injury beneath the surface of the skin

Chapter 2

WHAT IS
A PRESSURE ULCER?

A pressure ulcer is an area of injury to the skin and possibly the tissues beneath the skin as a result of pressure, or pressure along with shear and/or friction. The injury is usually situated over a **bony prominence**. Other names for a pressure ulcer are decubitus ulcer, pressure sore or bed sore

Pressure ulcers occur far too often in health care settings. A review of the prevalence over a ten year period in the U.S. was 10 to18% in acute care, 2.3 to 28% for long term care, and 0 to 29% for home care. Previous studies found the overall prevalence rate in Canadian health care settings to be even higher (26%). The difference may be partly due to the way in which the studies were done. About half of the pressure ulcers in the studies were stage 1 (skin was not broken).

Caring for people with pressure ulcers is expensive. The cost to heal a severe pressure ulcer may be $40,000 or more. The annual cost of pressure ulcer care in the U.S. has been estimated at between $5 and $8.5 billion. The cost in terms of human suffering cannot be measured. Pressure ulcers have a negative impact on a client's emotional, physical and social health. Financial costs to the sufferer and their family can be high. People lose independence and control. Pressure ulcers lead to longer hospital stays and increased **mortality**.

WHAT CAUSES PRESSURE ULCERS?

A pressure ulcer stems from pressure or pressure combined with **friction** or **shear**. Clients who are immobile (unable to move) are at increased risk because immobility leads to prolonged pressure. On average, a healthy individual changes position every 11.6 minutes. People who are unable to reposition themselves must rely upon caregivers to move them. When a person sits or lies in one position for a long time, the weight of the person's body presses on bone. The bone presses on the tissue and skin that cover it. The tissue is trapped between the bone and the bed or chair. This squeezes blood vessels in the skin and tissues, causing a reduced blood supply. A lack of nutrients and oxygen result and the tissue then starts to decay.

Friction and shear can also contribute to the creation of a pressure ulcer. Friction occurs when the skin rubs against something like a bed sheet, cast, or brace. Friction usually causes an injury, such as an abrasion, that you can see. Bony areas are more likely to be involved, such as the tailbone or ankles. This is especially true for people who have poor nutrition, for people who must be repositioned by others, and for older adults because their skin is usually thin and delicate.

Shear occurs beneath the surface of the skin as the result of a parallel force. For example, raising the head of the bed above 30 degrees will cause the resident to slide down the bed. When that happens, the skin sticks to the bed but the pelvis goes in the opposite direction. The same effect will occur when a person slides down in a chair. Tissue damage can occur.

There are two theories about how a pressure ulcer forms. One theory says that pressure ulcers form deep inside the tissue and move outwards. The second theory is that damage occurs from a skin injury on the surface that spreads to deep tissues. The most important thing to know is that, regardless of how they develop, pressure ulcers can be prevented. *It is much easier to prevent pressure ulcers than it is to cure them.*

We've discussed three forces - pressure, friction and shear – associated with pressure ulcers. Many other factors can also contribute to the development of pressure ulcers. These factors include:

Advanced age. The aging process causes changes to the skin. These changes make the skin less able to withstand normal wear and tear. The skin of older persons is more fragile. It is easily injured and it takes longer to heal.

Decreased skin sensation. When we sit in the same spot for a long time, the blood supply to that area is decreased. The decreased blood supply caused by pressure results in pain. Pain causes us to move, thus relieving the pressure. Clients with decreased sensation may not be able to feel the pain. They may stay in the same position much too long. A pressure ulcer may result.

Certain conditions such as **spinal cord injury, diabetes mellitus, stroke,** and **hypotension** can cause pressure ulcers.

Decreased nutrition or poor fluid intake.

Moist skin due to incontinence, excessive sweating, wound drainage or increased sweating from a high temperature

Products that irritate the skin.

Decreased mental status. Clients with decreased mental status may be unable to properly care for themselves.

Light skin coloring.

Smoking.

The use of certain drugs such as **steroids.**

Underweight or overweight. People who are either obese or very thin are at greater risk.

Of all the factors associated with the development of pressure ulcers, "pressure" is the most important. A small amount of pressure for a long period of time can do just as much damage as a great deal of pressure over a short period of time.

CONSIDER FOR A MOMENT ...

Think about the person you are caring for.

Which of these risk factors could apply?

RISK ASSESSMENT

How do you decide who is at risk for developing pressure ulcers? Different assessment tools (e.g. Braden, Norton, Waterlow, Gosnell) have been used to evaluate the risk of pressure ulcers for clients. The Braden Scale is used in many facilities in the U.S. and Canada.

The Braden Scale assesses the risk of pressure ulcer development based upon six risk factors – ability of the person to move, ability of the person to walk, sensation, friction and shear, moisture and nutrition. A scoring system is used to find out the level of risk that is present. The lower the score, the greater the risk:

Score on the Braden Scale	Level of Risk
15-18	At Risk
13-14	Moderate
10-12	High
9 or Lower	Very High

The Braden Scale is completed on admission and every three months afterwards in some health care facilities. In others, the assessment is done much more often. Hospitals and institutions have policies related to who should do the assessment and how often it needs to be done.

The Braden Scale helps determine the risk of pressure ulcer development so that steps can be taken to help prevent them. Clinicians need to evaluate the findings and decide what changes need to take place to prevent pressure ulcers. You may be asked to make changes to the care you give a person based on the findings from the Braden Scale.

CONSIDER FOR A MOMENT ...

Has the Braden Scale

(or similar risk assessment tool)

been completed on the

person you are caring for?

If so, how often is the assessment done?

Who is assigned to complete the assessment?

Chapter 3

SIGNS OF A
PRESSURE ULCER

The first sign of a pressure area is often a reddened area over a bony prominence. The reddened area will not go away even the pressure is relieved (e.g. the person is repositioned). There may be other symptoms, such as pain or a difference in temperature when compared to the surrounding area. The injured area may be warmer or cooler, firmer or softer than the surrounding skin. There could be burning, itching or tingling in the area.

It is difficult to detect the early stages of a pressure ulcer in persons with dark skin. The damaged area may appear to be a different color than the surrounding skin.

The more advanced pressure ulcers can involve breakdown of the skin, the tissues that lie below the skin and even the bone. There may be drainage from the ulcer. Skin can actually decay with severe pressure ulcers.

Pressure ulcers are usually found on bony prominences. A bony prominence is an area where the bone sticks out. Bony prominences are also called pressure points because they bear the weight of the body when a person is sitting or lying down.

The most common location for a pressure ulcer in adults is the coccyx or sacrum. The heel is the second most common site. Pressure ulcers, however, can be found in other parts of the body including the elbows, shoulder blades, hips, knees, ankles, toes or ear lobes. Pressure areas can also develop where two bony surfaces, such as the knees and ankles, rub together. In obese persons a pressure area can develop from the friction of skin rubbing against skin (e.g. under the breasts).

CONSIDER FOR A MOMENT ...

Think of a client who has had a pressure ulcer. What were the symptoms that you noticed?

STAGING

A pressure ulcer can range in severity from a minor injury that does not cause a break in the skin to a deep injury affecting muscle and sometimes even bone. Pressure ulcer development can be broken down into four stages based on the degree and depth of the injury:

Stage I

This is the stage with the least serious injury. The skin remains unbroken in this stage. There is redness in a localized area, usually situated over a bony prominence.

The color does not revert to normal when the pressure is relieved (e.g. the person is turned). If the person has a dark skin tone, the color of a stage 1 ulcer may appear to be different from that of the surrounding skin. The damaged area may feel firmer or softer than the skin next to it. It may also be a different temperature than the surrounding area.

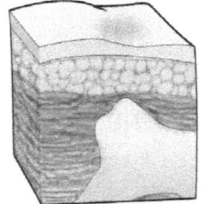

Stage II

The skin is broken although the wound is not deep. May appear as a shallow ulcer. There could be a blister which is either intact or broken.

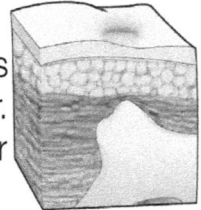

Stage III

This is a deeper injury. The tissue below the skin may be exposed although bone, tendon or muscle will not be visible. There may be some drainage. In locations where there is not much subcutaneous tissue, such as the earlobe or the bridge of the nose, the stage III ulcer will be shallow.

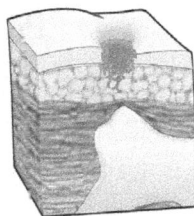

Stage IV

A very deep injury exposing bone, tendon or muscle. Drainage or eschar (a dry crust) may be present. If the ulcer involves the bone, the injury is more serious. Again, in areas with little or no subcutaneous tissue, the stage IV ulcer can be shallow.

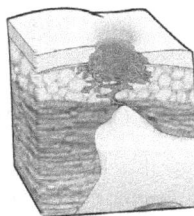

Unstageable

Some pressure ulcers are labelled as unstageable. These injuries are hidden by dead tissue or a dry crust, making it difficult to determine the exact extent of the injury. The injury could be either a stage III or a stage IV.

CONSIDER FOR A MOMENT ...

Are you caring for someone with a

pressure ulcer now? If so, do you know

if the ulcer is in stage I, II, III or IV?

PREVENTING PRESSURE ULCERS

Pressure ulcers are very costly and time-consuming to heal. A deep pressure ulcer can take many months to heal. It is far easier to prevent a pressure ulcer than it is to heal one.

Good Skin Care

One of the best things you can do to help prevent pressure ulcers is to take good care of the person's skin. Identify people who are at risk for developing pressure ulcers. Inspect their skin, especially bony areas, during baths and whenever they are positioned. Observe closely for common signs of a pressure ulcer. Never massage the skin over bony areas. Never massage an area that may be a pressure ulcer. Doing so could worsen the injury. Notify the appropriate health care professional if you observe symptoms of a pressure ulcer.

Check the care plan before you begin the person's bath. Older adults tend to have dry skin. The person you are caring for may not require a full bath every day. As well, he or she could be sensitive or even allergic to certain common products. When you bathe someone, clean the skin with a soft cloth or sponge and a mild cleansing agent (if used) to prevent injury or irritation. Avoid hot water. Pat, don't rub, the skin dry after the bath. Use a moisturizing cream to avoid dry skin. Apply the moisturizing cream to dry areas such as the elbows, legs and feet. Pay particular attention to the ankles and heels. Avoid alcohol-based skin products.

Aim to keep the skin dry. Skin may be moist from bladder or bowel incontinence, wound drainage or perspiration. People with urinary incontinence should have a thorough physical examination by a knowledgeable doctor. Urinary incontinence can usually be cured, treated, or successfully managed.

Incontinence exposes the skin to moisture and bacteria. It increases the chance of skin breakdown. Cleanse and dry the skin as soon as possible after an episode of incontinence and apply a moisture barrier as indicated on the care plan. A variety of incontinence products may be used. These products come in many sizes and absorbencies. They are designed to meet the needs of a variety of people at different times of the day or night. Ensure that you use the correct product for the correct time of day.

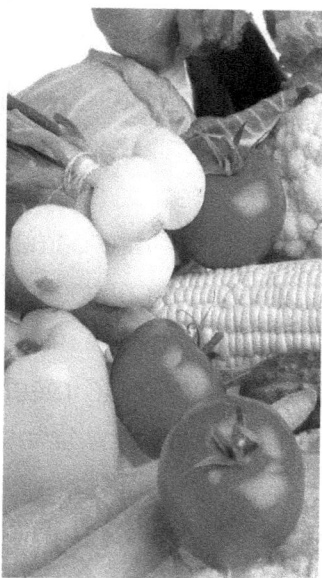

Nutrition

Adequate protein and other nutrients are essential to maintain healthy skin. An adequate fluid intake is also important. Encourage the person in your care to eat a healthy diet. Offer fluids throughout the day to prevent dehydration. Monitor their food and fluid intake. A healthcare professional should be notified if there is any concern about nutrition.

Chapter 4
POSITIONING

It is important to position people correctly and to ensure that their position is changed regularly. Proper positioning makes people feel more comfortable. It also helps with breathing and promotes blood circulation. Proper positioning techniques, along with regular position changes, help prevent pressure ulcers and contractures.

Some people are able to position themselves. Others will need your assistance. To properly position a person, you will have to assist him to turn from side to side or to move up in the bed. Due to their mental or physical condition, some people will not be able to assist at all with position changes.

- Ensure that you follow good body mechanics as you perform these procedures. Body mechanics refers to moving your body efficiently and safely. Using proper techniques will prevent injuries to yourself and the person in your care.

- Reposition the person regularly. It is generally recommended that people who cannot move on their own be turned and positioned every two hours. A two-hour turn schedule will work well for many people, but it may not meet the needs of everyone. So follow the care plan for your particular person to ensure that individual needs are met.

- Use pressure management devices as ordered for all the surfaces that may come into contact with the person's skin while sitting or lying down. Different types of mattresses, including foam, gel, air or fluid, have been used for this purpose. Special cushions are also available for wheelchairs or chairs to reduce pressure on the client's skin.

- Encourage people who are in a sitting position – either in a chair, a bed or a wheelchair – to change position every 15 minutes, even if only slightly. The person can lean over to shift the weight from one side to the other. Encourage as much activity as the person can tolerate.

- Avoid the use of donut-shaped (ring) cushions when seating someone. They have been found to reduce blood flow and cause swelling. They can actually increase the risk of pressure ulcers and should never be used.

- Plan what you are going to do and gather the items you will need before you position the person

- Ensure the privacy of the person you are caring for.

- Inform the person about the move that is to be made.

- If the person can assist with moving or repositioning in the bed, encourage him/her to do so as per the care plan.

- Follow the care plan and recommendations about lifting, transferring and positioning . Many organizations follow a "no lift" policy that stipulates that a mechanical lift must be used to lift people. It is often recommended to get help when positioning a person. Lift teams are regularly used in many health care facilities.

- Use a lift sheet to prevent friction and sheer injuries when moving a person up in bed or turning the person to the side. A lift sheet can be a drawsheet or a cotton sheet folded in half. Place it under the person so that it extends from under the head to just above the knees. Some facilities use a turning pad in place of a sheet or drawsheet. Remember to ask for advice or help with positioning as needed. Avoid dragging people up in the bed.

- Ensure that the bed is clean, dry, and unwrinkled. Wrinkles or damp sheets increase the risk of pressure ulcers developing.

- Use protective devices, such as a bed cradle, heel elevators, elbow protectors, pillows and foam wedges as ordered to relieve pressure. These devices are used for comfort as well as to protect bony prominences from coming in contact with one another. For example, a pillow placed between the knees can prevent pressure from the knees rubbing against each other when the person lies on the side.

- Ensure that the person's limbs and joints are properly positioned and supported (good body alignment). Gather all pillows, rolls and other equipment that you will need before you move the person. Pay particular attention to a paralysed limb. The person will have decreased sensation in this limb. Support the paralysed limb on a pillow to prevent injury and swelling.

- When you have finished positioning the person in your care, ensure that the call bell, if used, is within reach.

Wheelchair users

Wheelchair users have special concerns which you should be aware of. These include:

- Has the person been trained and can she perform self repositioning such as "roll", "forward lean" and "lift off"?

- Has an appropriately trained individual assessed the person's needs for seating?

- Have the family and caregiver been informed of the importance of repositioning every 15 minutes?

- Is the person using any prescribed pressure redistributing cushion? These cushions are available in foam, oil based, gel and dynamic (also called alternative or active).

- You should be aware that cushion covers may also be recommended for transfer, incontinence, body heat or other reasons.

- You should understand that the best seated posture is that which does not impede a person's ability to carry out any activities he wishes to perform.

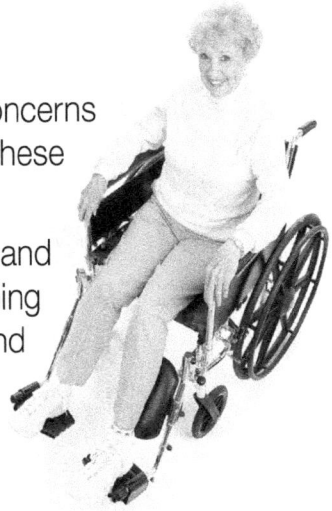

GOOD BODY MECHANICS

Good body mechanics include:

- Planning your move. Think about what you want to do and how you will do it. Will you need to ask others to help you? Will you need to use a lift?

- Position yourself close to the object you wish to move.

- Assume a wide stance and bend your knees before you begin your move.

- Avoid stretching, reaching, or twisting your body.

- Keep your abdominal muscles tight and tuck in your pelvis before moving an object.

- Hold objects as close as possible to your center of gravity when moving or carrying them.

- Avoid lifting. Instead, push, slide, roll, turn or pull objects.

CASE EXAMPLE

Mr. Horton is an 82-year-old resident in a nursing home. Mr. Horton has diabetes mellitus. He also had a stroke several months ago that left him with right-sided weakness. Mr. Horton cannot move about in the bed without assistance. He has difficulty swallowing and is incontinent of urine.

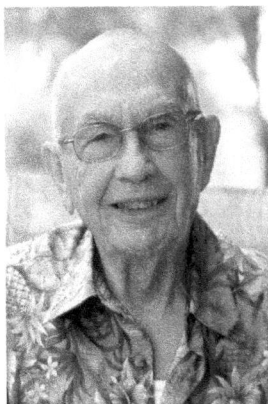

How many risk factors for pressure ulcers can you identify?

What signs and symptoms of pressure ulcers should you be observing for?

What can you do to help prevent pressure ulcers?

SUGGESTED ANSWERS TO CASE EXAMPLE

How many risk factors for pressure ulcers can you identify?

Mr. Horton has several risk factors for pressure ulcers. These include immobility, advanced age, diabetes mellitus, stroke and incontinence. Since Mr. Horton has difficulty swallowing he may be at risk for poor nutrition and inadequate fluid intake.

What signs and symptoms of pressure ulcers should you be watching out for?

You should look for a reddened area over a bony prominence. This is often the first sign of a pressure area. The injured area may be warmer or cooler, firmer or softer than the surrounding skin. The person may feel pain, burning, itching or tingling in the area. If Mr. Horton has dark skin, the damaged area may appear to be darker than usual or a different color than the surrounding skin.

What can the caregiver do to help prevent pressure ulcers?

Mr. Horton needs help to move about in bed. You will have to reposition Mr. Horton and provide good skin care to protect his skin from injury. Unless otherwise indicated on the care plan, you should reposition Mr. Horton every two hours or less. The skin (particularly the skin over bony prominences) should be inspected at each turn. He should be properly aligned with each positioning. The head of the bed should be kept at a 30° angle or less. A higher sitting position can be used if needed for brief periods only. A pressure-reducing mattress would be helpful.

Incontinence exposes his skin to moisture and to bacteria, which increases the risk of skin breakdown. The skin will have to be kept as dry and clean as possible.

Difficulty with swallowing may lead to poor nutrition and a lack of fluids. You should offer a healthy diet and extra fluids throughout the day. Mr. Horton's fluid and food intake should be monitored daily to ensure that it is adequate.

Chapter 5

POSITIONING IN BED

We've already discussed the benefits of regular positioning in the prevention of pressure ulcers. In some cases the physician orders specific positions because of the person's condition. When positioning the person in your care, consider his or her comfort and well-being. Pay particular attention to the pressure points. These are the areas at greater risk for pressure ulcers. Avoid positions that are not comfortable or, if you must use them, do so for short periods of time. Outlined below are several methods for positioning people in bed:

Supine

In the supine position, the person is positioned on the back. The head of the bed is flat.

- Place a small pillow under the head and shoulders
- Position the arms along the person's sides with palms facing down
- Place a small pillow under each arm and hand
- A small pillow or rolled towel can also be used for comfort as needed under the lower back,

next to each thigh to prevent the leg from turning outwards, under the thigh to keep the krees bent, or under the ankle. A **footboard** or rolled pillow can also be used to support the feet and prevent **footdrop**.

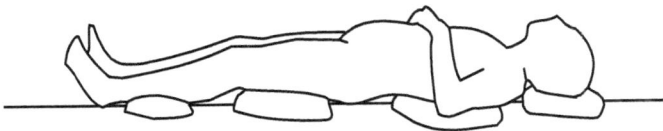

Supine Position

Prone

In the prone position, the person lies on the abdomen with the face turned to one side. This position is not recommended for someone with breathing problems. It can also cause pain for those with problems of the spine. It should only be used if indicated on the care plan and preferably for short periods of time.

- Ensure the bed is flat

- Place a small pillow under the head, abdomen and lower legs to prevent the toes from touching the bed

- Ensure the arms are bent

- Pressure areas may include the ear, chin, collarbones, elbows, knees, toes, genitalia for men, breasts for women.

Prone Position

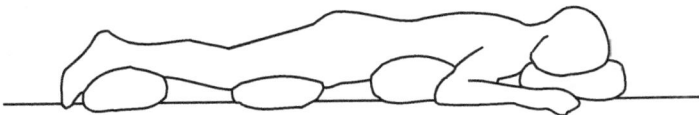

Fowler's

Fowler's position allows the person to sit up in bed. The head of the bed is raised from 45-60°. This position is helpful for people who have breathing problems and is often used when eating.

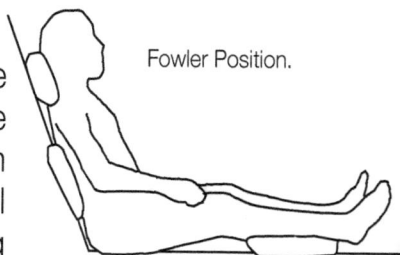

Fowler Position.

- Use one or more pillows behind the head, neck and upper back

- Use pillows to support the forearms and hands

- A small pillow or rolled towel can also be used for comfort as needed under the lower back, next to each thigh to prevent the leg from turning outwards, under the thigh to keep the knees bent, or under the ankle. A footboard or rolled pillow can also be used to support the feet.

- Pressure points include the heels, the sacrum and an area of the hip

Fowler's position puts significant pressure on the sacral area. As well, people often slide toward the foot of the bed, which can result in a shearing injury. To reduce the risk of a shear injury, keep the bed at 30° or less. This position is called "semi-fowler's". If you need to raise the head of the bed higher than this (for example to feed the person), do so for as short a time frame as possible.

Lateral

In the lateral position, the person lies on the side with most of the body weight resting on the hip and shoulder. All pressure is removed from the person's back.

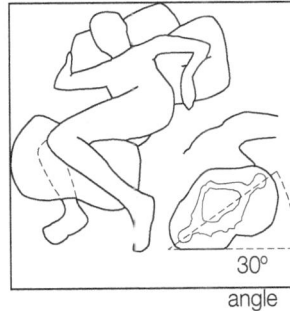

30°
angle

- Lower the bed to a flat position

- Position the person on the side

- Bend the lower leg slightly. Flex the upper leg more than the lower one.

- Flex both arms

- Position the lower shoulder forward.

- Use pillows for comfort and positioning. Place a small pillow beneath the head and neck, behind the back, and under the upper arm and leg.

- Pressure areas include the side of the head, the ear, shoulder, hip, knee and ankle.

Another common position is side-lying with the head of the bed at a 30° angle. A pillow goes under the person's head, shoulders and upper leg in this position. This position lifts up the hip to avoid putting pressure on it. This position has long been promoted as the position of choice for relieving pressure from most of the pressure points. Results from a recent study, however, found that this position may not be as effective as was previously thought. Some people found the position uncomfortable and the results were not any better than that of several other techniques. More research needs to be done into the area of positioning.

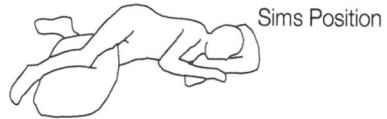
Sims Position

Sim's

The person is positioned towards the left and semiprone (almost lying on the stomach) while in this position. This position may be used when the person has to have an enema or some other procedure. Many older people find this position uncomfortable. Only use it when indicated on the care plan.

- Lower the bed to a flat position
- Position the client on the left side
- Place the left arm behind the person
- Flex the right arm more than the lower one
- Flex the left leg slightly
- Flex the right leg more than the left leg so that it does not lie on the lower leg
- Use a small pillow to support the head and neck
- Use pillows to support the upper arm and leg
- Pressure points include the ear, shoulder, hip, knee and ankle.

CONSIDER FOR A MOMENT ...

Imagine that you have to reposition someone who has been lying in the supine position. Identify four areas of the person's body that you should check for signs of a pressure ulcer.

CARING IN THE HOME

There are some special challenges to think about when you are caring for someone in the home. There may not be another caregiver present to help you. You may not have any special equipment to assist with body alignment. Beds may not be able to be raised and lowered. You must, however, still ensure the person's skin is well cared for and that he or she is properly positioned. You must still try to prevent pressure ulcers. Think about these issues before you go to the person's home. Consult with your supervisor. Some people do use mechanical lifts at home. In other cases, family members have been trained to assist with positioning people in bed.

Be creative as you plan how to position the person in your care. You may have to use towels, pillows, and blankets to maintain alignment. Refer to the care plan for positioning schedule and skin care routine. If you have any concerns or questions about the client's care, contact your health care professional.

USEFUL WEBSITES

Canadian Association of Wound Care: www.cawc.net

Canadian Association of Enterostomal Therapy: www.caet.ca

Registered Nurses Association of Ontario: www.rnao.org

Wound Ostomy & Continence Nurses Association:
www.wocn.org

National Pressure Ulcer Advisory Panel: www.npuap.org

The Wound Healing Society: www.woundheal.org

American Academy of Wound Management: www.aawm.org

Pressure Ulcer Awareness Program:
www.preventpressureulcers.com

International Wound Care Course (IIWC): www.twhc.ca

Body1.inc: www.wounds1.com

The Wound Care Information Network: www.medicedu.com

Association for the Advancement of Wound Care:
www.aawc1.com

Wound Care Institute: www.woundcare.org

World Wide Wounds: www.worldwidewounds.com

European Pressure Ulcer Advisory Panel: www.epuap.org

CONCLUSION

Pressure ulcers occur quite often in health care settings. They are costly to manage and have a negative impact on a person's health. They lead to longer hospital stays and increased mortality. The three main causes of pressure ulcers are pressure, friction and shear. Many other factors contribute to the development of pressure ulcers. Pressure ulcers are far easier to prevent than cure. With good skin care, proper nutrition and frequent positioning, most pressure ulcers can be prevented.

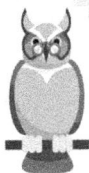

CHECK YOUR KNOWLEDGE

1. What are the risk factors of pressure ulcers?

2. What are the signs of a stage I pressure ulcer?

3. How can pressure ulcers be prevented?

4. Name three important points to know about positioning.

5. Describe the technique for positioning a person in a supine position.

TEST YOURSELF

Please circle to indicate the best answer:

1. The back-lying position is called:

a) Supine

b) Prone

c) Lateral

d) Fowler's

2. To provide good skin care, you should:

a) Aim to keep the skin dry

b) Massage all reddened areas

c) Use hot water to wash your clients

d) Give each client a full bath every day

3. While assisting someone to turn, you notice a reddened area over the hip. What should you do?

a) Ignore it

b) Gently rub the reddened area

c) Vigorously rub the reddened area

d) Notify the appropriate health care professional

4. What is often the first sign of a pressure ulcer?

a) A skin tear

b) Shallow ulcer with bruising

c) Drainage over a dark red area

d) Reddened area over a bony prominence

5. What are the pressure points for a person in Sim's position?

a) Ear, shoulder, hip, knee and ankle

b) Heels, sacrum, and an area of the hip

c) The side of the head, ear, shoulder, hip, knee and ankle

d) The back of the head, shoulder blades, sacrum, heels and elbows

6. Which risk factor for pressure ulcers is the most important one?

a) Pressure

b) Decreased nutrition

c) The use of certain drugs

d) Decreased skin sensation

7. What are the most common locations for pressure ulcers in adults?

a) Elbows and sacrum

b) Hips and the back of the head

c) Earlobes and heels

d) Coccyx and sacrum

ANSWERS

1. a) Supine is the correct term for lying on one's back.

2. a) It is important to ensure that perspiration, urine or anything out of the ordinary does not adversely affect the skin.

3. d) Notify the health care professional in order to prevent a pressure ulcer developing.

4. d) A reddened area is a major warning sign to get help immediately.

5. a) A diagram of the Sim's position will indicate these pressure points; usually, this is not the most comfortable position.

6. a) Pressure is always the most important factor, and is the key to preventing pressure ulcers.

7. d) The coccyx and sacrum are the most vulnerable areas, especially for people who use wheelchairs.

REFERENCES

Baldwin, K. (2006). Damage control: Preventing and treating pressure ulcers. Nursing Made Incredibly Easy! 4 (1), 12-26.

Baranonski, S. (2006). Raising awareness of pressure ulcer prevention and treatment. CE. Advances in Skin and Wound Care, 19, (7), 398-405.

Cuddigan, J, Berlowitz, D. and Ayello, E. (2001). Pressure ulcers in America: Prevalence, incidence and implications for the future. An Executive Summary of the National Pressure Ulcer Advisory Panel Monograph. Advances in Skin & Wound Care, 14 (4). Feature Article.

Hawkins, S., Stone, K., & Plummer, L. (1999). A holistic approach to turning patients. Nursing Standard, 14(3), 52-56.

Keast, D., Parslow, N., Houghton, P., Norton, L. and Fraser, C. (2006). Best practice recommendations for the prevention and treatment of pressure ulcers: Update 2006. Wound Care Canada, 4 (1), 31-43.

Kozier, B., Erb, G., Berman, A. J., & Burke, K. (2000). Fundamentals of nursing: Concepts, process, and practice (6th ed.). Upper Saddle River, NJ: Prentice Hall Health.

National Pressure Ulcer Advisory Panel (NPUAP) (2007). Retrieved February 20, 2007, http://www.npuap.org/documents/NPUAP2007_PU_Def_and_Descriptions.pdf

Niezgoda, J. & Mendez-Eastman, S. (2006). The effective management of pressure ulcers. Advances in Skin and Wound Care: The Journal for Prevention and Healing, 19, (1), Supplement, 3-15.

Sorrentino, S. (2004). Mosby's Canadian textbook for the support worker. Toronto, ON: Mosby.

Stegman, J. (2005). Stedman's medical dictionary for the health professions and nursing, Illustrated, 5th ed. New York: Lippincott Williams and Wilkins.

ALL ABOUT BOOKS

Trusted • Reliable • Certified

- 40+ titles available

- Comply with accreditation and regulatory bodies

- Suitable for caregivers, boomers with elderly parents, health workers, auxiliary health staff & patients

- Self study style with "test yourself" section

- Health On the Net (HON) certified

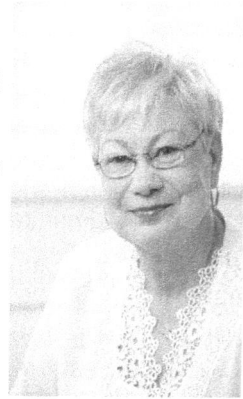

Some of our titles:

Alzheimers Disease	Arthritis	Multiple Sclerosis
Pain	Strokes	Elder Abuse
Falls Prevention	Incontinence	Nutrition & Aging
Personal Care	Positioning	Confusion
Transferring people	Care of the Back	Skin Care

For complete list of titles go to www.mediscript.net
Other websites:
www.woundcareclient.com www.allergyasthmaclient.com

Contact: 1 800 773 5088
Fax 1800 639 3186 • Email; mediscript@rogers.com